Overcome Life Circumstances

With the Word of God

Sharron Downs

Overcome Life Circumstances: With The Word of God
By Sharron Downs
Published by Sharron Downs
www.sharrondowns.info

Copyright

Amplified Bible Scripture quotations marked "AMP" are taken from the Amplified® Bible, Copyright © 1954, 1958, 1962, 1964, 1965, 1987 by The Lockman Foundation. Used by permission. www.Lockman.org

CEV Scripture quotations marked "CEV" are from the Contemporary English Version Copyright © 1991, 1992, 1995 by American Bible Society, Used by Permission.

ESV The Holy Bible: English Standard Version Scripture quotations marked "ESV" are from the ESV Bible® (The Holy Bible, English Standard Version®), copyright © 2001 by Crossway Bibles, a publishing ministry of Good News Publishers. Used by permission. All rights reserved.
http://www.crossway.org

Good News Translation Scriptures Quotations marked "GNB" or "GNT" are from the Good News Bible © 1994 published by the Bible Societies/HarperCollins Publishers Ltd UK, Good

News Bible © American Bible Society 1966, 1971, 1976, 1992. Used with permission.
http://www.biblesociety.org.uk

King James Version Scripture quotations marked "KJV" are taken from the Holy Bible, King James Version. Used by permission.

New American Standard Bible Scripture quotations marked "NASB" are taken from the New American Standard Bible®, Copyright © 1960, 1962, 1963, 1968, 1971, 1972, 1973, 1975, 1977, 1995 by The Lockman Foundation. Used by permission. www.Lockman.org

New International Version Scripture quotations marked (NIV) are taken from the Holy Bible, New International Version®, NIV®. Copyright © 1973, 1978, 1984 by Biblica, Inc.™ Used by permission of Zondervan. All rights reserved worldwide.
http://www.zondervan.com

New King James Version Scripture quotations marked "NKJV" are taken from the New King James Version. Copyright © 1982 by Thomas Nelson, Inc. Used by permission. All rights reserved.

New Living Translation Scripture quotations marked (NLT) are taken from the Holy Bible, New Living Translation, copyright © 1996, 2004, 2007 by

Tyndale House Foundation. Used by permission of Tyndale House Publishers, Inc., Carol Stream, Illinois 60188. All rights reserved.
http://www.newlivingtranslation.com/
http://www.tyndale.com

Scripture quotations marked "MSG" or "The Message" are taken from The Message. Copyright 1993, 1994, 1995, 1996, 2000, 2001, 2002. Used by permission of NavPress Publishing Group.http://www.navpress.com/

Contents

Title Page

Copyrights Page

Book Dedication

Introduction

- Life's Situations
- Decrees
- Overcome Life Circumstances
- Scriptures to Meditate
- Affirmations
- Words of Encouragement
- Conclusion
- Author
- Notes

Book Dedication

This book is dedicated to those who have had challenges, situations of hopelessness, disappointments, and mental instability. Whether you have been hurt by a dysfunctional family, bad relationships, or people who may have taken you for granted, there is hope. For anyone who has lived in a verbal abusive relationship or you may currently be dealing with this, there is hope. Whatever the situation or circumstance, you need a positive word of encouragement and redirection to see yourself in a better place. God's word will provide a way of escape. You no longer have to go through life alone.

God is so good and gracious. God just knows how to make everything better. I pray this book will be an inspiration to you. It's my prayer that you are able to relate and find some parallels which will truly inspire, help and bring clarity to areas where you were uncertain. Lastly, individuals and families who are searching for closure, trust God through his Word.

Introduction

Are you coping with a stressful situation, mental Instability, health concerns, or going through tough times? Let me encourage you. It may seem like there's no way out. You may not know what to do. You may know who to turn to. You may not know who you can trust. You may be living in fear. You may be angry or discouraged. You are not alone. Let me encourage you.

There is hope. You don't have to give up. There is mental stability in the word of God. There's peace in the word of God. There's hope in the word of God. Trust in the word of God, you no longer have to doubt or be angry. You no longer have to be misunderstood or feel abandoned. You no longer have to feel unworthy. You no longer have to have any uncertainty because God is here to help you.

God has blessed me to write this book during times of uncertainty, times of fear, times of loss, and times of negativity. God is our hope. We are living in an end time along with a life of daily uncertainties. Start to believe in yourself again. See things differently with an open mind, clear heart, positive words and things will begin to change. Pray about situations which you feel are out of control and you need help. God is so good and gracious He will send help.

This book is interactive. There are places to write your feelings, thoughts and emotions in the moment. There's also notes at the end of the book to keep all of your experiences so you'll see your growth and how you used to have those negative behaviors and now you are set free and delivered. Lastly, remember to write the dates next to everything, it helps you keep track of when it ended. Enjoy the process to a new level.

Feeling Discouraged

Do you feel stuck, heavy, sad, or hopeless? What does it mean for you to feel discouraged? What just happened recently in your life? What happened in the past which makes you feel discouraged, hopeless, sad, heavy, stuck or frustrated? What are some feelings or emotions which make you feel this way? Write them down, so later you will pray for these areas or emotions and find a scripture to help alleviate these feelings.

_____

_____

_____

Well, "You are not alone". You do not have to go through life feeling stuck, feeling sad, feeling discouraged, feeling hopeless, feeling like no one cares, and feeling like you do not matter. God knows you inside and out. God made you and formed you out of the dust of the ground. God is still the same God who was with Adam and Eve and He is with you today. God knew you and formed you in your mothers womb. God knows you inside and out. You have to trust God right now and let's read the scripture.

Psalm 34:17-18 GNT "The righteous call to the Lord, and he listens; he rescues them from all their troubles. The Lord is near to those who are discouraged; he saves those who have lost all hope."

Matthew 11:28 KJV "Come unto me, all ye that labour and are heavy laden, and I will give you rest."

I want you to write down how you're feeling.

_____

_____

_____

_____

1 Peter 5:6-9 KJV "Humble yourselves therefore under the mighty hand of God, that he may exalt you in due time: casting all your care upon him; for he careth for you. Be sober, be vigilant; because your adversary the devil, as a roaring lion, walketh about, seeking whom he may devour: whom resist stedfast in the faith, knowing that the same afflictions are accomplished in your brethren that are in the world."

Search the Scriptures and find verses that will help you with the feeling of discouragement, hopelessness and feeling stuck. Pray to God and call out each of the things you wrote and give it all over to God. Meditate the scriptures for comfort and relief. Give it all over to God. Once it's written down go not pick it back up.

There are several scriptures to help in any capacity of life. Reading scriptures and saying words of encouragement, prayers, positive affirmations, decrees and declarations will definitely make a difference in your life. Keep reminding yourself, you are not alone. God is here with you just like the Scripture says. If you are crying out for help, God is listening and he is ready to rescue you. Be encouraged. Pray and turn it all over to God.

Today start journaling, start writing down how you are feeling. (There is a section at the end of the book for even more note taking).

God is with you. God has you in His heart and mind. You are not alone. You don't have to listen to the negativity that's going on around you. God will help you. God is here. Scripture says, if your heart is broken, you'll find God right there. If you feel helpless, God is there, cry out to God, he will hear you, he will deliver you.

Solution:
Be very transparent, open and honest with yourself and write down your feelings and thoughts. Trust the process. The next step is to fall out of agreement with discouragement. You do this by speaking. You say, "I fall out of agreement with being discouraged".

Jeremiah 29:11 NKJV "For I know the thoughts that I think toward you, says the Lord, thoughts of peace and not of evil, to give you a future and a hope."

II Corinthians 12:9 NKJV "And He said to me, "My grace is sufficient for you, for My strength is made perfect in weakness." Therefore most gladly I will rather boast in my infirmities, that the power of Christ may rest upon me."

You will no longer be discouraged if you truly believe what you are saying and want change. You will focus on the things of God according to your faith be it done unto you. Say, "I am no longer engaging in discouragement", expect to see changes in your life where it pertains to discouragement.

Psalm 55:22-23 MSG "Pile your troubles on God's shoulders— he'll carry your load, he'll help you out. He'll never let good people topple into ruin. But you, God, will throw the others into a muddy bog, Cut the lifespan of assassins and traitors in half. And I trust in"

Feeling Heartbroken

What does it feel like to be brokenhearted? Do you feel like it's a lot of emotional or physical pain? Do you feel extremely stressed? How are you coping with the broken heart? Do you feel like your heart has fallen out of your body? Do you feel grief? Do you feel pain?

Psalm 34:18 MSG "If your heart is broken, you'll find God right there; if you're kicked in the gut, he'll help you catch your breath."

Maybe, you feel like Jeremiah in this scripture: . .Jeremiah 8:18 NLT "My grief is beyond healing; my heart is broken."

Take a moment to write down your thoughts.

_____

_____

_____

_____

The feelings you are feeling, let's recognize where they initiated. Let's look deeper to see if it is from a relationship or something else that led you to the feeling of being brokenhearted? Was it a loss of a loved one, a bad relationship, how are you coping through these days, these moments of the feeling of a broken heart? (Write down your feelings)

By writing your feelings down it helps to see and release your words of brokenness to receive your breakthrough.

The feelings you have are real and you want to address them. You will find comfort. God knows your feelings, God knows everything about it and God is here to help you. You are not alone, you are chosen for this very hour. Think about the things you have tried in the past, see if they line up with the scriptures. I challenge you to find other scriptures. Look for scriptures to help overcome obstacles and situations you're currently struggling with. Here are a few scriptures to help in this area of brokenness.

Psalms 147:3 NLT "He heals the brokenhearted and bandages their wounds."

1 Peter 5:7 AMP "casting all your cares [all your anxieties, all your worries, and all your concerns, once and for all] on Him, for He cares about you [with deepest affection, and watches over you very carefully]."

Psalms 34:18 NLT "The Lord is close to the brokenhearted; he rescues those whose spirits are crushed."

Deuteronomy 31:8 AMP "It is the LORD who goes before you; He will be with you. He will not fail you or abandon you. Do not fear or be dismayed.""

Isaiah 61:1 NLT "The Spirit of the Sovereign Lord is upon me, for the Lord has anointed me to bring good news to the poor. He has sent me to comfort the brokenhearted and to proclaim that captives will be released and prisoners will be freed."

Solution:
I say to you, be strong and courageous, do not be terrified, dismayed, or intimidated, for the Lord your God is with you wherever you go. You no longer have to have feelings of a broken heart. God mends broken hearts. Take this time today and write down your feelings, be open and honest, transparent with yourself and God.

_____

_____

_____

_____

_____

Allow yourself to be healed from the feeling of a broken heart. Take your time to heal. Do not worry. Allow God to show you how to move to the next step. God will send the right people to help you through this situation. Whether it was from a loss of a loved one or loss of a bad relationship, God's love for you will heal the broken heart. It will help you go to your next, you have to trust God and know this season in your life is only temporary.

2 Corinthians 4:16-18 AMP "Therefore we do not become discouraged [spiritless, disappointed, or afraid]. Though our outer self is [progressively] wasting away, yet our inner self is being [progressively] renewed day by day.

For our momentary, light distress [this passing trouble] is producing for us an eternal weight of glory [a fullness] beyond all measure [surpassing all comparisons, a transcendent splendor and an endless blessedness]! So we look not at the things which are seen, but at the things which are unseen; for the things which are visible are temporal [just brief and fleeting], but the things which are invisible are everlasting and imperishable."

So we're not giving up. It may seem like things are falling apart on the inside. God is making all things new. There's not a day which goes by without his unfailing grace.

Read these scriptures along with others to help get rid of life's problems and situations you are experiencing right now.

Lord, I'm asking you to please remove all of their feelings of being broken-hearted. Whatever they are experiencing, all of the feelings they've had and all the people who have broken their heart, forgive them. I ask you, Lord right now enter into their heart. Let them fall out of agreement with being brokenhearted and recognize they no longer need to live with this feeling of brokenness. They are healed, set free and delivered.

Proverbs 13:12 MSG "Unrelenting disappointment leaves you heartsick, but a sudden good break can turn life around."

Ephesians 6:13-18 MSG "Be prepared. You're up against far more than you can handle on your own. Take all the help you can get, every weapon God has issued, so that when it's all over but the shouting you'll still be on your feet. Truth, righteousness, peace, faith, and salvation are more than words. Learn how to apply them. You'll need them throughout your life. God's Word is an indispensable weapon. In the same way, prayer is essential in this ongoing warfare. Pray hard and long. Pray for your brothers and sisters. Keep your eyes open. Keep each other's spirits up so that no one falls behind or drops out."

Feeling Angry

Are you feeling angry or you feeling irritated? Are you feeling frustrated? Do you have a lot of pent-up emotion that's causing you to feel angry, about a particular situation or circumstance, you can't control? Right now, pause, breathe and read the scripture for encouragement.

Philippians 4:6 NLT "Don't worry about anything; instead, pray about everything. Tell God what you need, and thank him for all he has done."

1 Peter 5:7 NLT "Give all your worries and cares to God, for he cares about you."

Proverbs 15:1 NLT "A gentle answer deflects anger, but harsh words make tempers flare."

_____

_____

_____

How often do you experience anger issues? Do you always experience mood swings and act out with anger? Do you know when you start to feel angry or do people have to bring it to your attention? Do you have people saying, what's going on, you seem angry? Do you raise your voice at others when you are in a conversation? Are you aware of what triggers your anger? Is it also caused by something that's going on in your environment or something that happened in your past and you feel you cannot control? Pray and ask God to reveal it to you. Write down your thoughts and feelings.

_____

_____

_____

_____

_____

Ephesians 4:31 NLT "Get rid of all bitterness, rage, anger, harsh words, and slander, as well as all types of evil behavior."

Ephesians 4:26 GNT "If you become angry, do not let your anger lead you into sin, and do not stay angry all day."

Psalm 4:4-5 MSG "Complain if you must, but don't lash out. Keep your mouth shut, and let your heart do the talking. Build your case before God and wait for his verdict."

Solution:
So here are some things to do to ensure if you start to feel angry you do not sin. Breathe: pause, let's reevaluate the situation. Is it worth it to become angry and use negative energy on that person or situation? No stop using a lot of negative energy on either that person or the situation. Just breathe, relax and say you need a minute, say nothing else walk away if needed. Remember you are the one who wants to be

better and not go down to their level. You need to react the opposite of what they think you will do. Do not give into their ways.

Psalms 37:8 NLT "Stop being angry! Turn from your rage! Do not lose your temper— it only leads to harm."

Keep in mind some people will try to have you become angry on purpose, meaning sometimes people push those trigger points on purpose to get you angry and out of character. Keep in mind you don't have to act out with anger. Choose positive words, no more negativity. If someone hurts, irritates or says something wrong to you, stay in peace, walk away. Tell them that's bothering you. Say to that person stop saying that or stop doing that and if you're able to walk away and move yourself from that situation by all means gain peace. Do not allow yourself to become irritated. Speak what you want to happen. Use positive affirmations and words to change your life. Don't curse yourself or put anything else negative on you like anger. You will be better. See things the way God sees you.

Proverbs 19:11 NLT "Sensible people control their temper; they earn respect by overlooking wrongs."

That was one perspective to help you think about your anger. Start writing it down, journaling the days and times that brought you to that anger and see if you can start to illuminate those things, those places, those thoughts and those situations which are causing you to become angry.

_____

_____

_____

Another way to change the situation is to start singing a song to change your atmosphere. It works because you change your mindset and take your mind off anger and into the words of the song. It works. What's your favorite song? What song makes you happy? Sing it.

Ephesians 4:26 NLT "And "don't sin by letting anger control you." Don't let the sun go down while you are still angry,"

James 1:20 CEV "If you are angry, you cannot do any of the good things God wants done."

James 1:19 NLT "Understand this, my dear brothers and sisters: You must all be quick to listen, slow to speak, and slow to get angry."

Angry feelings are negative feelings. This takes up too much energy to be angry. When you have these feelings take a moment and breathe, step away if you can and gain control of your thoughts and emotions. Eliminate circumstances that hinder you. Be free. God is here to help you. Call out to God for help immediately when you feel anger.

Scripture tells us how we need to handle anger. Let God guide you and help you.

First you must stop doing anything immoral or evil. Instead, be humble and accept the message planted in you to save you. Decree: you will fall out of agreement with anger in the name of Jesus. You no longer want to be angry. Ask the Lord to remove these feelings of anger from you according to the scriptures and by faith it will be done for you. Release love in those areas where anger and hate may reside.

Proverbs 14:29 NLT "People with understanding control their anger; a hot temper shows great foolishness."

Feelings of Resentment

Do you find yourself holding grudges, acting jealous, feeling bitter about job security about something that somebody has done to you? How do you react when you're with other people during the holidays? What triggers your need to feel bitter? Do you want to remain bitter? Why are you holding grudges? Why are you jealous? What are you jealous about? What causes your bitterness? Are you always sarcastic? Do you have feelings of bitterness toward a person because of a bad relationship? Bitterness is about hate and anger.

If you answered yes, there may be several different reasons.

First, here is a scripture to help.

Hebrews 12:14-17 MSG "Work at getting along with each other and with God. Otherwise you'll never get so much as a glimpse of God. Make sure no one gets left out of God's generosity. Keep a sharp eye out for weeds of bitter discontent. A thistle or two gone to seed can ruin a whole garden in no time. Watch out for the Esau syndrome: trading away God's lifelong gift in order to satisfy a short-term appetite. You well know how Esau later regretted that impulsive act and wanted God's blessing—but by then it was too late, tears or no tears."

Write down this week every time that you feel bitter about a particular situation, circumstance, person, conversation, television show. Whatever the case is whenever you have these feelings of bitterness, I want you to write it down and see if you could have handled the situation differently.

_____

_____

_____

_____

_____

What was the first thing that you did when you noticed that you had feelings of bitterness?

Let's look at what the Bible says about bitterness.

Ephesians 4:31 is another good one that we've already covered for bitterness. Let's stop being bitter, angry and mad at others. Don't yell at anyone or curse each other or even be rude.

Ephesians 4:31 AMP "Let all bitterness and wrath and anger and clamor [perpetual animosity, resentment, strife, fault-finding] and slander be put away from you, along with every kind of malice [all spitefulness, verbal abuse, malevolence]."

Proverbs 20:22 CEV "Don't try to get even. Trust the Lord, and he will help you."

James 3:14 CEV "But if your heart is full of bitter jealousy and selfishness, don't brag or lie to cover up the truth."

Ensure that you have conquered and been delivered from this before you move onto the next. I do realize some of these feelings you may be experiencing are related to other feelings. If this is your case make sure you pair those with their counterparts. Speak positive words and meditate on scriptures which I reference to help you will help you be delivered from that particular feeling of negativity.

Solution:

There are so many scriptures and there's so many ways to overcome but you have to be open, you have to be willing to allow God to change your heart. You need to be able to change your mindset because if you can change your mindset you won't have these negative feelings occurring all the time. You will have these strategies to replace those negative words with positive words. God is definitely positive and we all know that the devil is the one that brings these negative feelings, negative issues and all of these things that are evil.

Matthew 6:12 AMP "And forgive us our debts, as we have forgiven our debtors [letting go of both the wrong and the resentment]."

There are many ways to get rid of the negativity. The easiest way is through words. Speak better, speaking positive affirmations and have a positive mindset. You have to trust God, be very transparent with yourself and allow yourself to be open. You do not want to be vulnerable to others but open to yourself in your own quiet time so that you can get the deliverance that you need. You want the help that I am providing to you through scripture, decrees, words and affirmations.

Say, "I fall out of agreement with bitterness in the name of Jesus". Say it from your heart and the Lord will help you with your bitterness. Words are powerful. Say, " Lord take it away." You no longer want it. You will no longer entertain anything that is not from God. Lord according to our faith be it done unto us from this day forward, We will no longer act in bitterness. Amen

Ephesians 4:27 AMP "And do not give the devil an opportunity [to lead you into sin by holding a grudge, or nurturing anger, or harboring resentment, or cultivating bitterness]."

Proverbs 3:5-12 MSG "Trust God from the bottom of your heart; don't try to figure out everything on your own. Listen for God's voice in everything you do, everywhere you go; he's the one who will keep you on track. Don't assume that you know it all. Run to God! Run from evil! Your body will glow with health, your very bones will vibrate with life! Honor God with everything you own; give him the first and the best. Your barns will burst, your wine vats will brim over. But don't, dear friend, resent God's discipline; don't sulk under his loving correction. It's the child he loves that God corrects; a father's delight is behind all this."

Feeling Rejected

Feelings of rejection, well this one is huge. I know lots of people who have gone through this. I went through this as well. I can probably say that almost everybody in their lifetime has gone through the feeling of rejection. What really is rejection?

Rejection is like pushing someone away. These emotions can be painful. Rejection from a loved one, a parent or somebody at school. Rejection from a friend, a relationship, a job there are so many areas not in our life where you can feel rejected but it's how you deal with it. It's being able to recognize that you are being rejected and how to deal with it. Once you see it you want to change that situation immediately. So many times people do not even realize that they are suffering from the spirit of rejection. People continue on and on until they can't handle it anymore.

Let's take a moment to reflect a time or current situation where you had these feelings of rejection. What are your thoughts? How did you cope?

Luke 20:17 AMP "But Jesus looked at them and said, "What then is [the meaning of] this that is written: 'THE [very] STONE WHICH THE BUILDERS REJECTED, THIS BECAME THE CHIEF CORNERSTONE'?"

Jesus himself was even rejected and so looking at that particular scripture in Luke it let us know how Jesus handled himself because everything that we're going through Jesus actually went through. This a perfect example of how we should live by searching the Scriptures and finding out how Jesus handled himself is going to be easy right? I know not necessarily. Do you have to be able to relate the Scriptures? You have to be able to understand the Scriptures, put it into your own lifestyle; which is why I would highly recommend finding a Bible that speaks in today's language. The message translation (MSG) or the CEV brings things to practical purposes and you are able to understand what's really going on.

2 Corinthians 12:9 GNT "But his answer was: "My grace is all you need, for my power is greatest when you are weak." I am most happy, then, to be proud of my weaknesses, in order to feel the protection of Christ's power over me."

John 1:11 GNT "He came to his own country, but his own people did not receive him."

1 Peter 5:8-9 "Be alert, be on watch! Your enemy, the Devil, roams around like a roaring lion, looking for someone to devour. Be firm in your faith and resist him, because you know that other believers in all the world are going through the same kind of sufferings."

And just as we've done in previous situations, write down your feelings. Make sure you are journaling your feelings, your thoughts, which made you feel rejected. Let's start to knock those walls down of rejection, so you will be able to love again; you will be able to trust again; and you won't have these other feelings of bitterness or anxiousness. You will feel better about yourself. Speak, "I am no longer rejected in Jesus name. I fall out of agreement with rejection in Jesus' name so be it unto me".

Solution:

If Jesus was rejected and he was the Son of God. You are in good company- if they did it to Jesus they will do it to you. Do as he did to help overcome the struggles of rejection. We have all experienced this. This typically occurs at work or from family. Let the rejection no longer hinder you. Recognize you have hurt and rejection in your heart towards a person, company, family members etc. let them go. You need freedom. No longer will you be bound by rejection from this day forward. You are set free and delivered from rejection. Thank God for healing you.

1 Thessalonians 5:9-11 MSG "God didn't set us up for an angry rejection but for salvation by our Master, Jesus Christ. He died for us, a death that triggered life. Whether we're awake with the living or asleep with the dead, we're alive

with him! So speak encouraging words to one another. Build up hope so you'll all be together in this, no one left out, no one left behind. I know you're already doing this; just keep on doing it."

No one wants to experience a feeling of rejection. They hurt and if you continue to rehearse them over and over in your mind it will become a hindrance and you do not need any hindrances. Life has enough going on by itself. Let's look at a few scriptures to help in times of rejection.

John 5:43 NLT "For I have come to you in my Father's name, and you have rejected me. Yet if others come in their own name, you gladly welcome them."

1 Timothy 4:4 AMP "For everything God has created is good, and nothing is to be rejected if it is received with gratitude;"

Feeling Misunderstood

Do you ever have feelings of being misunderstood? Do you think about what you want to say before you speak?

If you answered yes, do you feel people do not understand you? Do they see you as different? Have you always had a feeling of being set apart?

Do you act differently or are you unique? Have you ever had anyone call you weird? Do you feel that people just don't accept you because you are different ? How does that make you feel? What type of feelings do you have or can express being misunderstood? If you can relate, stop and write out exactly how you are feeling.

Take this time and write down the feelings you are feeling and express them in the journal pages in the back of the book. Let's journal them and figure out the root cause of this feeling of being misunderstood.

_____

_____

_____

Let's look at the Scriptures and see what God has to say about being misunderstood.

II Corinthians 1:12-14 NKJV "For our boasting is this: the testimony of our conscience that we conducted ourselves in the world in simplicity and godly sincerity, not with fleshly wisdom but by the grace of God, and more abundantly toward you. For we are not writing any other things to you than what you read or understand. Now I trust you will understand, even to the end (as also you have understood us in part), that we are your boast as you also are ours, in the day of the Lord Jesus."

Let's capture the very essence of God. Definitely fall out of agreement with the feelings and the spirits that are attached to this so that you can gain total deliverance in every area of your life.

I can say feelings of being misunderstood have absolutely nothing to do with you. You are unique and others do not know how to communicate with you. They see you as "weird" because you are different. You are not weird, you're on a different higher level than they are. Your thoughts are creative, innovative, and unique. You see things in pictures and can relate to simple things and talk in mysteries. This is how it was with Jesus, Joseph, Daniel, Samuel and Abraham in the Bible. You are in good company. Continue your uniqueness! Live who you are called to be, you have purpose on the inside of you. You were created for greatness, do not come down to their level, bring them up to yours or keep it moving, (there used to be a phrase "get to steppin" . You will not allow them to talk to you in any type of way and you shouldn't).

Solution:

Keep your head high and speak words of greatness. You are unique, use your voice and speak positive affirmations about your uniqueness. Have faith, high self esteem, great expectations and continue to see yourself as God sees you, like a diamond a cut above an Ambassador of the Kingdom of God.

Here is a scripture to sum up this situation.

1 Corinthians 12:1-3 MSG "What I want to talk about now is the various ways God's Spirit gets worked into our lives. This is complex and often misunderstood, but I want you to be informed and knowledgeable. Remember how you were when you didn't know God, led from one phony god to another, never knowing what you were doing, just doing it because everybody else did it? It's different in this life. God wants us to use our intelligence, to seek to understand as well as we can. For instance, by using your heads, you know perfectly well that the Spirit of God would never prompt anyone to say "Jesus be damned!" Nor would anyone be inclined to say "Jesus is Master!" without the insight of the Holy Spirit."

Feeling Lonely

What does it mean to feel lonely? Are you experiencing some times of loneliness now? What feelings are you experiencing?

Psalms 68:6 AMP "God makes a home for the lonely; He leads the prisoners into prosperity, Only the stubborn and rebellious dwell in a parched land."

I'm sure many of you can relate to this situation as we were all going through this in 2020. Did you experience days, months, weeks of loneliness as a result of the COVID 19 pandemic?

Isaiah 41:10 NKJV "Fear not, for I am with you; Be not dismayed, for I am your God. I will strengthen you, Yes, I will help you, I will uphold you with My righteous right hand.'"

Did you feel like you had no one to turn to? Were you in a home alone and you couldn't wait to get outside but then when you did you were nervous? Were you scared, felt afraid?

What exactly caused the loneliness to get worse?

_____

_____

_____

Did you have extreme moments of loneliness? Did you want to reach out to someone but don't know how?

What level of loneliness are you experiencing on a level of 1 to 5 where five is extreme?

_____

_____

_____

_____

Explain the symptoms that you are experiencing and what makes you think that you are lonely?

_____

_____

_____

_____

_____

Did someone make you feel this way or tell you that's what's going on in your life? What causes these bouts of loneliness? Have you always isolated yourself from others? Do you feel better alone rather than being around people? Write down your thoughts.

_____

_____

_____

_____

_____

Deuteronomy 31:6, 8 NKJV "Be strong and of good courage, do not fear nor be afraid of them; for the Lord your God, He is the One who goes with you. He will not leave you nor forsake you." And the Lord, He is the One who goes before you. He will be with you, He will not leave you nor forsake you; do not fear nor be dismayed.""

Loneliness is real. Your feelings are real and this is very serious. Take a minute to breathe.

Breathe in, breathe out. Relax, pause for a minute.

Now say "I am not lonely, I am not alone" Jesus is here with me I am not alone".
(Say this as often as needed)

Joshua 1:9 NKJV "Have I not commanded you? Be strong and of good courage; do not be afraid, nor be dismayed, for the Lord your God is with you wherever you go.""

Psalms 25:16-17 NKJV "Turn Yourself to me, and have mercy on me, For I am desolate and afflicted. The troubles of my heart have enlarged; Bring me out of my distresses!"

Solution:

Philippians 4:11-13 AMP "Not that I speak from [any personal] need, for I have learned to be content [and self-sufficient through Christ, satisfied to the point where I am not disturbed or uneasy] regardless of my circumstances. I know how to get along and live humbly [in difficult times], and I also know how to enjoy abundance and live in prosperity. In any and every circumstance I have learned the secret [of facing life], whether well-fed or going hungry, whether having an abundance or being in need. I can do all things [which He has called me to do] through Him who strengthens and empowers me [to fulfill His purpose—I am self-sufficient in Christ's sufficiency; I am ready for anything and equal to anything through Him who infuses me with inner strength and confident peace.]"

Repeat this out loud a few times until your mindset changes and you start feeling better and loneliness starts to dissipate.

Continue saying positive affirmations and build up your faith and confidence. Jesus is here. You are uniquely loved and will never live another day of loneliness again. If it tries to come to your mind, tell it to leave and don't accept it. This will be a process, do not give up, be persistent. You control your feelings and emotions from this point on. Jesus will help you. Pray call on God to make things better. Speak what you want to happen and watch God work it out . All this is through powerful word confessions!

Write in this book (notes section) what you are now feeling and experiencing. No more feeling lonely, sad, disappointed, low self-esteem, feeling alienated, alone like no one cares.

Isaiah 41:10 GNT "Do not be afraid—I am with you! I am your God—let nothing terrify you! I will make you strong and help you; I will protect you and save you."

John 16:32 GNT "The time is coming, and is already here, when all of you will be scattered, each of you to your own home, and I will be left all alone. But I am not really alone, because the Father is with me."

Ecclesiastes 4:9 CEV "You are better having a friend than to be all alone, because then you will get more enjoyment out of what you earn."

God is here to make all things better. You are definitely better than when you started reading this section! Receive your deliverance right now let's fall out of agreement with loneliness and say that you will never be lonely another day in your life. You gave your life to God.

God is your only source. Establish that relationship with God and the feelings of loneliness are going to subside daily. Continue to write down your feelings each and every time you start to have that feeling of self worthlessness and the feeling of loneliness. You are not alone. God is here, God is with you, trust God, rely on God to make all things better, release happiness and joy into your life right now; and know that loneliness cannot stay when the Spirit of God and the fruits of the spirit are living within you.

Repent, ask God for forgiveness and to come into your heart. Say Lord live in me and through me from this day forward Lord I belong to you. I believe you died, rose again on the third day and took away all my sins. I belong to you."

If you just spoke this aloud. . Welcome into the kingdom of God. Loneliness was nailed to the cross and you don't have to feel lonely; you will never be alone when you have Jesus as your

Lord and Savior! Fall out of agreement with loneliness and say I am loved, happy not sad, above only never beneath.

Feeling Sick

Did the doctors give you a bad report? What makes you feel like you have symptoms of sickness? Is sickness all in your mind? Are you constantly saying you are sick? Do you agree with the doctor's reports? Did the doctor give you a long list to confess because of your family history? Well, you do not have to accept it. They may have had those diseases but it can stop with you. No sickness or disease shall come near you. Take a moment to write down what the doctor said, this way you will be able to come back to this moment and see what it was which was spoken over you and you did not agree with but gave it over to the Lord in prayer. You have the realization no sickness or disease shall come near you.

_____

_____

_____

_____

Speak the word of God over your situation. Watch how the Word of God goes to work on your behalf. Read these scriptures twice a day Morning and night. Let the scriptures be your medicine. Take as directed. (more if needed for pain)

Psalms 91:3, 6, 10, 14-16 CEV "The Lord will keep you safe from secret traps and deadly diseases. And you won't fear diseases that strike in the dark or sudden disaster at noon. and no terrible disasters will strike you or your home. The Lord says, "If you love me and truly know who I am, I will rescue you and keep you safe. When you are in trouble, call out to me. I will answer and be there to protect and honor you. You will live a long life and see my saving power.""

Why do you think that you are sick?
If you are saying, this is you and you are feeling sick; having symptoms of sickness in your body; stomach hurt and you feel sick emotionally? Breathe and let's not focus on the symptoms because these are subject to change. Today will

be your last day to confess sickness. No more sickness in your body.

Solution:

Philippians 4:6-8 NKJV "Be anxious for nothing, but in everything by prayer and supplication, with thanksgiving, let your requests be made known to God; and the peace of God, which surpasses all understanding, will guard your hearts and minds through Christ Jesus. Finally, brethren, whatever things are true, whatever things are noble, whatever things are just, whatever things are pure, whatever things are lovely, whatever things are of good report, if there is any virtue and if there is anything praiseworthy—meditate on these things."

Question, was Jesus ever sick? Then as a child of God you do not have to be sick either. Start to speak healing over your body believing God is your healer.

1 Peter 2:24 GNT "Christ himself carried our sins in his body to the cross, so that we might die to sin and live for righteousness. It is by his wounds that you have been healed."

James 5:14-15 GNT "Are any among you sick? They should send for the church elders, who will pray for them and rub olive oil on them in the name of the Lord." "This prayer made in faith will heal the sick; the Lord will restore them to health, and the sins they have committed will be forgiven."

Everyone let me tell you, you do not have to be sick or accept or allow sickness to enter your body. I know that sounds totally different from what you have been "taught". Sickness is of the devil and it's a curse. You can speak to it and it has to leave your body in the name of Jesus.

The Bible says by Jesus stripes you are healed. Jesus died on the cross and bore all of our sicknesses and diseases and nailed them to the cross so all you have to do is claim your healing no more sickness. When you speak faith filled positive words, speak words of life no more sickness. Speak words of life no more death. Let your words be your confession to your health. If the doctor gives you a report, do not agree with him. I know that's not me, I don't have that. Be bold God will honor your faith. Refuse to accept the negative report no matter what it may look like. Stand in faith, quote the scriptures and say by Jesus stripes I'm healed. Sickness cannot live on or in your body. You will not allow sickness, not even a headache allergy nothing. You are delivered from any firm of sickness from this moment forward.!

If you happen to go to the doctors and they ask you about your family history you have "none", I repeat you have "zero" of those "family symptoms or diseases' ' you do not have a history of any of those symptoms. Do not speak sickness or disease over you or your family. They will try to put it on you with their words, do not accept it "refuse the negative report." Your family is perfectly healthy. Your ancestors and immediate family are healthy. No sickness or disease in your family line.

The Bible says, if you are sick or if there are any sick among you, let them contact the elders of the church. Let them lay hands on you and you shall recover.

I repeat, say "you do not agree with sickness of any type mentally, physically, emotionally, internally, absolutely no sickness". You do not have to agree with them. Look at it this way, they are only "practicing medicine". General practitioner, (generally practicing on you, when you tell them your symptoms, they have to look it up and diagnose you according to what the computer or book says). I know you've seen this at doctors offices.

James 5:14 CEV "If you are sick, ask the church leaders to come and pray for you. Ask them to put olive oil on you in the name of the Lord. If you have faith when you pray for sick people, they will get well. The Lord will heal them, and if they have sinned, he will forgive them."

Hebrews 4:12-13 CEV "God's word is alive and powerful! It is sharper than any double-edged sword. His word can cut through our spirits and souls and through our joints and marrow, until it discovers the desires and thoughts of our hearts. Nothing is hidden from God! He sees through everything, and we will have to tell him the truth."

3 John 1:2 KJV "Beloved, I wish above all things that thou mayest prosper and be in health, even as thy soul prospereth."

Isaiah 53:5 AMP "But He was wounded for our transgressions, He was crushed for our wickedness [our sin, our injustice, our wrongdoing]; The punishment [required] for our well-being fell on Him, And by His stripes (wounds) we are healed.

Feeling Abandoned

Do you have or ever have you ever had feelings of abandonment? Do you seek to please others more than yourself? Do you always give, give, give and never receive? In your relationships are you pushing others away to avoid rejection? Do you feel the need for codependency? What makes you feel abandoned? Were you abandoned as a child?

If you happened to answer yes to all of the above, take a moment now and write your thoughts down. I know it may be painful but this is a part of the healing process.

_____

_____

_____

_____

Let us go through this situation and see what solutions we can find to assist and end this feeling of abandonment.

We found out it was indeed a generational situation that took place, where you were left behind. Now you feel insecure, always withdrawn, stay to yourself.

If you answered yes to any of those, let's take a moment and start journaling right now. Write down what makes you feel abandoned, how you feel in that situation, when did you start feeling this; was it again in your childhood with your mother? Was it perhaps with your father? Was it with another loved one? Did it just happen? Write everything down... take your time, no rush. It's very important to be able to recognize these feelings and be open, honest and very transparent with yourself.

Solution:
I want you to say that you fall out of agreement with the feeling of abandonment, you will no longer want to feel abandoned, you no longer want to feel unworthy, you no longer want to be left behind, you no longer want to have this

feeling of loss! You no longer want to become dependent upon anyone but God going forward! Lord, I give all of these feelings over to you now. I no longer want them and I know you will remove them once I confess it and give it to you.

1 Peter 5:7 AMP "casting all your cares [all your anxieties, all your worries, and all your concerns, once and for all] on Him, for He cares about you [with deepest affection, and watches over you very carefully]."

Say, "you will have good relationships, you will not look to others to validate you". Say, "you will no longer have abandonment issues; you curse abandonment at the root in Jesus name".

Now let's look at a few scriptures that will help us go through the need of being delivered from abandonment .

Psalm 27:10 "Although my father and my mother have abandoned me, Yet the LORD will take me up [adopt me as His child]."

Right now let's fall out of agreement with abandonment and know that you are accepted by God. You no longer have to accept abandonment, you are free and delivered as long as you please God that's all that's necessary. God first in everything you do. I rejoice with you on your deliverance. Remain free.

Feeling Hopeless

Are you feeling hopeless, sad, or unhappy? Are you feeling like you have no possible solution to make things better? Do you have feelings of uncertainty? Do you have certain situations that make you feel like you want to give up hope? Do you have moments where you cry uncontrollably for no reason?

How long have you been having these feelings of hopelessness? Is it to the point of depression, lack of self-worth, lack of self-esteem? What is causing you to feel hopeless right now? Is it a relationship?

_____

_____

_____

Romans 15:13 AMP "May the God of hope fill you with all joy and peace in believing [through the experience of your faith] that by the power of the Holy Spirit you will abound in hope and overflow with confidence in His promises."

Psalm 69:17 AMP "Do not hide Your face from Your servant, For I am in distress; answer me quickly."

Psalm 86:1 AMP "Incline Your ear, O LORD, and answer me, For I am distressed and needy [I long for Your help]."

1 Corinthians 10:13 GNT "Every test that you have experienced is the kind that normally comes to people. But God keeps his promise, and he will not allow you to be tested beyond your power to remain firm; at the time you are put to the test, he will give you the strength to endure it, and so provide you with a way out."

Solution:
Jeremiah 29:11 ESV "For I know the plans I have for you, declares the Lord, plans for welfare and not for evil, to give you a future and a hope."

Start writing down all of your feelings for this situation. Before you move onto the next situation, make sure you have surrendered all those feelings over to God and you no longer have these feelings (remember it's a process). If you're going through this again or it happens to come back up, remember you know the scriptures to go to. You know how to search the Scriptures to find peace. You have tools in that particular area, then fall out of agreement with the things that are not of God. These are solutions which can be used in every area of your life. I want you to remember the steps, principles, solutions and strategies. I want you to be successful for the rest of your life. I want the peace of God to be with you.

Feeling Guilty

Have you ever had a feeling of guilt? Have you ever hurt somebody or did something wrong which made you feel like you were causing some form of guilt to someone?

If you answered yes, it made me feel guilty, violated, lying, cheating, stealing all of this made me feel guilty.! Write your feelings here.

_____

_____

_____

I'm sure each of us have had all these feelings. You may have experienced these and you need to be able to forgive yourself and stop having these feelings of guilt. Therefore let's right now take the time to write down in our journal the things that make you feel guilty that you have done in the past or current. Say, "Lord forgive me I repent of (all the things you wrote down) guilt in each of the areas I've mentioned or your words you say on your own. "

_____

_____

_____

Let's write down what triggers you to feel this way?

_____

_____

_____

_____

_____

_____

What did you do to change the situation, if you changed it? What plans are you going to do to change the situation so that it does not happen again? Do you understand what guilt is? What makes you think that you even have a feeling of guilt? How long have you had these feelings?

_____

_____

_____

_____

Let these solutions you write down help you. If whatever you did worked, great now, I'll give you scriptures and solutions to keep them from reoccurring.

Solution:

God has forgiven us of all of our sins. We need to forgive ourselves, forgive those who we have sinned against; so we do not have these feelings of condemnation, guilt, pain and negativity. All of these things that keep coming up in your mind the devil wants you to rehearse over and over in your mind. No stop! Now we have to fall out of agreement with guilt, fall out of agreement with anxiety and everything that attaches itself to the feeling of guilt! Fall out of agreement with guilt whether it's from an influence from another person, something on television, something you did online, something you said, something or someone.

If you made somebody feel a certain way you can also experience the feeling of guilt. Forgive yourself now. Say I forgive myself from (fill in the blank) "_____" whatever it was. No more condemnation. Let's look up some scriptures we can associate these feelings with so that we can no longer have the feeling of guilt or shame. You can only say and believe in your heart all guilty sins, transgressions are gone and you are no longer that person people want to keep bringing up. Once you are born again the old man is erased. You are a new creature in Christ.

Job 33:9 NIV "'I am pure, I have done no wrong; I am clean and free from sin."

Romans 8:1 NIV "Therefore, there is now no condemnation for those who are in Christ Jesus,"

Romans 10:9 NIV "If you declare with your mouth, "Jesus is Lord," and believe in your heart that God raised him from the dead, you will be saved."

Galatians 6:4 GNT "You should each judge your own conduct. If it is good, then you can be proud of what you yourself have done, without having to compare it with what someone else has done."

Feeling Neglected

Are you feeling neglected? Have you ever felt neglected? What makes you feel that you are being neglected?

We have all been there. Let's face it we need to get rid of these feelings of being neglected and ignored. These feelings are real. emotionally do you feel this was portrayed in your relationships with loved ones? Do you give people the silent treatment as a part of being neglected? Have you been abused? Do you feel traumatized by some feelings of neglect? Was it intentional?

_____

_____

_____

_____

Let's deep dive into these feelings with the Word of God, so that we can get to the root cause of the feelings of being neglected and then we will be able to see what God has to say in his word.

Solution:

Numbers 6:24-26 GNT "May the Lord bless you and take care of you; May the Lord be kind and gracious to you; May the Lord look on you with favor and give you peace."

Genesis 1:27 KJV "So God created man in his own image, in the image of God created he him; male and female created he them."

Feeling Weak

Have you ever had a feeling of being weak, not strong, not in control of your feelings ? Have you had feelings of being tired, fatigue, overwhelmed, feeling like this is too much? What about lack of confidence which makes you feel weak? Feelings of not being strong or bold? Are you looking at yourself against someone else to feel that you are weak in an area?

If you answered yes to those, let's journal now and figure out what causes you to feel weak.

_____

_____

_____

Why do you think you were not strong? Why do you think that you were not bold? What is the main reason for the weakness? Has someone told you you're weak?

What makes you feel you are not strong or confident or self-aware in a particular area? Did this happen when you were at work, felt incompetent against your peers? Did you feel that you didn't get a job because you were weak? Was it a leadership issue? Write your responses here.

_____

_____

_____

_____

_____

So many questions. They may not all pertain to you or you may have several other situations. Either way, Let's start to fall out of agreement with the feeling of being weak.

Stand up look in the mirror Say aloud:

- ☐ " I am strong"
- ☐ "I will never be weak another day in my life"
- ☐ " I will never lack another day in my life"
- ☐ "I am courageous"
- ☐ "I am victorious"
- ☐ " I am bold"
- ☐ "I believe, God has given me strength to overcome every obstacle"

What are some affirmations which come to your mind to help you when you feel weak?

_____

_____

_____

_____

_____

Solution:

Use your voice, speak words of faith, affirmations, decrees to overcome negativity.

Fall out of agreement with everything that is not of God. Right now see yourself as God sees you. We are all created in the image of God. Have faith in God to know you are strong in every area of your life. You will no longer be seen as weak. Do not accept it from anyone. Don't be self conscious or self sabotage yourself another moment. You are not weak. You are strong. You are a wonderful person, an overcomer, intelligent, strong and blessed. Your voice matters. Start speaking these strategies to unlock your full potential!

2 Corinthians 12:9-10 NLT "Each time he said, "My grace is all you need. My power works best in weakness." So now I am glad to boast about my weaknesses, so that the power of Christ can work through me. That's why I take pleasure in my weaknesses, and in the insults, hardships, persecutions, and troubles that I suffer for Christ. For when I am weak, then I am strong."

Ephesians 6:10 AMP "In conclusion, be strong in the Lord [draw your strength from Him and be empowered through your union with Him] and in the power of His [boundless] might."

2 Chronicles 15:7 MSG ""But it's different with you: Be strong. Take heart. Payday is coming!""

Feeling Controlled

Do you ever have Feelings like you are being controlled by someone? Every time you think you're getting ready to do something that person tells you no, you are to do what they want you to do and their way is the only way.

Are you feeling controlled in a relationship, are you feeling controlled by parents, by your spouse, by your boss, your best friends, anyone other than God? We are only to be controlled by God and the Holy Spirit . No human flesh should control us especially if it is in the negative.

Are they controlling you to do things that are against your will? Do you start to feel uncomfortable, overwhelmed, have feelings of doubt, self worthlessness or even have low self-esteem? What do you do?

_____

_____

Solution:

I am here to help. I'm letting you know that God is here to send deliverance to you. He will help you every step of the way. When we trust in God, we will cast all of our cares upon him because he cares for us. This scripture is a very appropriate scripture. It helps us. This scripture is real. The Holy Spirit is here to help, guide, comfort us. Think of it as we are being led by the Holy Spirit in Christ Jesus.

What a joy, hallelujah. Let's take that leap of faith and start allowing the Holy Spirit to speak to us, to lead, guide and help us walk each day filled with God's love and God's original plan and a purpose for our life.

Philippians 4:7 GNT. "And God's peace, which is far beyond human understanding, will keep your hearts and minds safe in union with Christ Jesus."

John 14:25-27 MSG ""I'm telling you these things while I'm still living with you. The Friend, the Holy Spirit whom the Father will send at my request, will make everything plain to you. He will remind you of all the things I have told you. I'm leaving you well and whole. That's my parting gift to you. Peace. I don't leave you the way you're used to being left—feeling abandoned, bereft. So don't be upset. Don't be distraught."

Psalm 56:1-4 MSG "Take my side, God—I'm getting kicked around, stomped on every day. Not a day goes by but somebody beats me up; They make it their duty to beat me up. When I get really afraid I come to you in trust. I'm proud to praise God; fearless now, I trust in God. What can mere mortals do?"

Feeling Fearful

Are you feeling fearful? Do you have more fear or anxiety than you do faith or trust in yourself? What is causing these feelings of fear? Ate the feelings of fear from work, family, financial, mental or all of the above?

We do not have to live in fear. For God did not give us a spirit of fear but of power, love and a sound mind. 2 Timothy 1:7 AMP "For God did not give us a spirit of timidity or cowardice or fear, but [He has given us a spirit] of power and of love and of sound judgment and personal discipline [abilities that result in a calm, well-balanced mind and self-control]."

We need to rely on God to help us. Challenge: take each day by day and let's deal with those fears head-on. Let's talk about what fears you may have so that we can pray and have deliverance in those areas of fear, for we do not have to have fear. God is not to be afraid of, God is love!

Job even said it in his book, the very thing that I feared that's what came up on me.

Job 3:25 NKJV
"For the thing I greatly feared has come upon me, And what I dreaded has happened to me."

From this moment forward refuse to fear anything else. ladies and gentlemen let's trust in God for deliverance. let's break the strongholds whether they're generational, relationships, soul ties, let's break all this fear.

With God all things are possible. We don't have to live in fear another moment, hour, day, week or ever again.

Matthew 19:26 NKJV "But Jesus looked at them and said to them, "With men this is impossible, but with God all things are possible.""

What are some things that cause fear? What are some things which make you feel fearful or even makes you uncomfortable?

_____

_____

Solution:

Let's search the scriptures and see what God has to say about fear. I guarantee you after the session you will no longer walk in fear. We will pray the prayer of faith, you will be delivered and set free once and for all. To God be the glory, so be it unto you according to your faith amen.

II Timothy 1:7 NKJV "For God has not given us a spirit of fear, but of power and of love and of a sound mind."

Isaiah 41:10 AMP "Do not fear [anything], for I am with you; Do not be afraid, for I am your God. I will strengthen you, be assured I will help you; I will certainly take hold of you with My righteous right hand [a hand of justice, of power, of victory, of salvation].'"

1 John 4:17-18 MSG "God is love. When we take up permanent residence in a life of love, we live in God and God lives in us. This way, love has the run of the house, becomes at home and mature in us, so that we're free of worry on Judgment Day—our standing in the world is identical with Christ's. There is no room in love for fear. Well-formed love banishes fear. Since fear is crippling, a fearful life—fear of death, fear of judgment—is one not yet fully formed in love."

Psalms 56:3 AMP "When I am afraid, I will put my trust and faith in You."

Feeling Burdened

What is it to feel burdened? What makes you think that you are a burden? Have you ever felt burdened way down, like life is just being sucked out of you and you feel weighted, tired and dismayed? Where did you turn? What did you do to change that feeling?

Well, Jesus died on the cross for our sins he bore all of us sicknesses, diseases and all of our burdens. We don't have to worry about anything we don't have to fear. We don't have to have anxiety. We don't have to feel weighed down, tired or dismayed. Give it over to God.

What are the symptoms you are feeling which makes you feel burdened? Do you feel like you can't go on anymore, you're so tired? Hope is in the way. No more being burdened. Father God, remove these feelings, emotions and thoughts of burdensome worry from them right now. Worry burdens I command you to go now in Jesus name. Get out and leave them you have no right in them and the blood of Jesus covers them right now. Lord, we thank you and consider it done in Jesus name. Amen

Write down any feelings and thoughts you are experiencing. Let's try to put those feelings into words so God can give you direction and you receive total deliverance from burdens now.

_____

_____

_____

_____

Solution:

God, I ask you to give them peace of mind. Start to change our mindset and really trust and rely on God who is the author and finisher of our faith. Open your heart and allow God to heal your heart and remove all burdens now.

Psalms 55:22 AMP "Cast your burden on the LORD [release it] and He will sustain and uphold you; He will never allow the righteous to be shaken (slip, fall, fail)."

Isaiah 41:10 NKJV "Fear not, for I am with you; Be not dismayed, for I am your God. I will strengthen you, Yes, I will help you, I will uphold you with My righteous right hand.'"

Psalms 68:19 GNT "Praise the Lord, who carries our burdens day after day; he is the God who saves us."

Feeling Stressed

Are you feeling stressed? How many times have we heard this? How many times have we felt this? Stress is definitely real. Stress needs to be dealt with and not tolerated.

You may be going through this right now. For most of the nation in 2020 this was definitely in the top 3 "STRESS" but it does not have to continue to be on your radar. I'm here to let you know you do not have to live in stress. You do not have to have anxiety. The scriptures tell us to "cast all of our cares over to God for he cares for us".

1 Peter 5:7 AMP "casting all your cares [all your anxieties, all your worries, and all your concerns, once and for all] on Him, for He cares about you [with deepest affection, and watches over you very carefully]."

We will trust in the Lord with all our heart and lean not unto our own understanding. This is the only way to have God as our only source in every area of our lives.

Proverbs 3:5-7 AMP "Trust in and rely confidently on the LORD with all your heart And do not rely on your own insight or understanding. In all your ways know and acknowledge and recognize Him, And He will make your paths straight and smooth [removing obstacles that block your way]. Do not be wise in your own eyes; Fear the LORD [with reverent awe and obedience] and turn [entirely] away from evil."

Solution:

Now let's tackle some of the feelings which make you feel stressed and let's dive into what the trigger points are of certain words, phrases, images you may encounter.

Do you feel stressed when you watch the news? Do you feel stressed when you go to work? Do you feel stressed when driving in traffic? Do you feel stress with your children? Do you feel stress in your marriage? What else causes you stress?

Take a moment to write them down. I want you to be able to know exactly when the stressful situations were lifted. I want you to see your progress and know exactly when you conquered that particular stressful situation, be sure to include the date it happened. Rejoice and celebrate, thank God for removing that stress.

_____

_____

_____

Also write it down to become aware of the feelings and come to know the "trigger points" to avoid so you will make sure not to have this added stress in your life.

_____

_____

_____

_____

The Bible says that we can overcome all things through Christ who strengthens us. I guarantee you, you will no longer have to live in stress once God rebukes the devourer for your sake.

Right now wherever you are, fall out of agreement with stress once and for all. Say, "Lord, I give this situation and circumstance over to you. I fall out of agreement with stress and I fall into agreement with peace for my life." "Devil you will not cause me to have fear about anything because Greater is He that's in me than he that's in the world. No weapon formed against me shall prosper. God is for me and I refuse to have stress, anxiety or anything that is not from God, in and on my life. I am delivered and set free!" Amen, Amen and Amen. Thank you, Lord.

We believe all of the symptoms and manifestations that fall in the line of stress are no longer holding you bound. You are delivered. You are set free. The curse has been reversed. Let those who love courses receive it on to themselves. God's got you. From this moment on, trust and believe God to remove all stressful situations, circumstances and possibly even people, if they try to return.

Revisit this situation and solution as often as needed. Take your time, it's a process. Asking God for deliverance will come now with a sincere heart and determination to be set free.

Matthew 11:28-30 MSG ""Are you tired? Worn out? Burned out on religion? Come to me. Get away with me and you'll recover your life. I'll show you how to take a real rest. Walk with me and work with me—watch how I do it. Learn the unforced rhythms of grace. I won't lay anything heavy or ill-fitting on you. Keep company with me and you'll learn to live freely and lightly.""

Psalms 55:22 AMP "Cast your burden on the LORD [release it] and He will sustain and uphold you; He will never allow the righteous to be shaken (slip, fall, fail)."

Romans 8:31-39 MSG "So, what do you think? With God on our side like this, how can we lose? If God didn't hesitate to put everything on the line for us, embracing our condition and exposing himself to the worst by sending his own Son, is there anything else he wouldn't gladly and freely do for us? And who would dare tangle with God by messing with one of God's chosen? Who would dare even to point a finger? The One who died for us—who was raised to life for us!—is in the presence of God at this very moment sticking up for us. Do you think anyone is going to be able to drive a wedge between us and Christ's love for us? There is no way! Not trouble, not hard times, not hatred, not hunger, not homelessness, not bullying threats, not backstabbing, not even the worst sins listed in Scripture: They kill us in cold blood because they hate you. We're sitting ducks; they pick us off one by one. None of this fazes us because Jesus loves us. I'm absolutely convinced that nothing—nothing living or dead, angelic or demonic, today or tomorrow, high or low, thinkable or unthinkable—absolutely nothing can get between us and God's love because of the way that Jesus our Master has embraced us."

Start to live day by day starting to write things down in your journal each and every time you feel stress. Let's conquer them immediately if the enemy tries to come into your mind and tell you other than what you know the word of God. Review the scriptures and this section on this strategy to overcome STRESS. Remember to speak: you say I fall out of agreement with stress, I trust God, the Holy Spirit is our comforter He will help you.

I believe God with you for your deliverance. You will be set free once and for all in Jesus name so be it onto you Amen. God's word will never return void.

Feelings of Doubt

Have you ever had feelings of doubt? Do you doubt the things that you are capable of doing in the kingdom of God? What are some things that cause doubt in your life right now? Do you doubt that you are a good parent? Do you doubt that you are a good spouse? Do you doubt that you are a good person? Do you doubt God?

_____

_____

_____

_____

Solution:
Matthew 11:28-30 NKJV "Come to Me, all you who labor and are heavy laden, and I will give you rest. Take My yoke upon you and learn from Me, for I am gentle and lowly in heart, and

you will find rest for your souls. For My yoke is easy and My burden is light."

Right now, let's face your doubt. Read what the scriptures tell us.

Isaiah 41:10 NKJV "Fear not, for I am with you; Be not dismayed, for I am your God. I will strengthen you, Yes, I will help you, I will uphold you with My righteous right hand.'"

Are you saying, "I can't do this, I can't do that, I'm not able to do this, I'm not able to do that, I won't do this?

Eliminate doubt, no more discouragement, no more negative feelings. No longer allow the enemy to entrap your mind with feelings of doubt, discouragement or feelings of being dismayed. God has made each of us in his own image and likeness. We are sons and daughters of the Most High and Holy God. Therefore, God's spirit is in you. God does not have doubts so therefore you will not have any doubts either. I say to you, resist the devil and he will flee from you. PERIOD..... When these feelings come to your mind, fall out of agreement with them, ask God for help immediately! Continue to confess all doubt is removed, eliminated and out of your life according to His will plans and purpose for your life! Expect your situation to change.

II Corinthians 9:8 NKJV "And God is able to make all grace abound toward you, that you, always having all sufficiency in all things, may have an abundance for every good work."

Philippians 2:12-13 MSG "What I'm getting at, friends, is that you should simply keep on doing what you've done from the beginning. When I was living among you, you lived in responsive obedience. Now that I'm separated from you, keep it up. Better yet, redouble your efforts. Be energetic in your life of salvation, reverent and sensitive before God. That energy is God's energy, an energy deep within you, God himself willing and working at what will give him the most pleasure."

Feeling Unheard

We all have a voice and we all want to be heard one way or another, which way are you seeking?

Are you seeking to be heard in a marriage, are you seeking to be heard to your parents, are you seeking to be heard by children?

What is it you want people to hear from you? How are you voicing your opinion with things? Are you putting them on social media? Are you drawing? Are you painting?

Why do you feel that you are not being Heard? Let's examine some situations in which you feel unheard. Is it because of the environment you are currently in or is it because of everything that's going on in the world right now that makes you feel unheard?

_____

_____

_____

Do you ever think about if Jesus was unheard when he was ministering during the time he was here on the earth? Jesus would always decree a thing, cast things out that were not right, and anything not pleasing to God the Father. Let's follow the example of Jesus and start to take our authority back. Let's use our authority the way God intended. If we are in God's likeness and His image we should do as God did in every area of our lives.

Solution:

Speak and meditate this scripture: Ecclesiastes 2:12 KJV "And I turned myself to behold wisdom, and madness, and folly: for what can the man do that cometh after the king? even that which hath been already done."

Think of it like this. Everything we are to do on this earth has already been done. God created the world one time and all plans, purposes, visions, instructions were given to us at birth! They are all inside of us. They have been birthed and breathed in us. This is why we live from the inside out as children of the Most High

God. We are created in His image. Pause and think and meditate on this. It takes a minute to comprehend. Another way to see this is we are just walking through life's "play scene "according to the way it was already predestined when God made us and conformed us in our mother's womb. We have a voice we will be heard! Make sure you do it God's way (kingdom of God) and his glory will be established.

Let's speak the words of God, speak peace, speak joy, speak love, speak happiness, speak healing, speak and create your world God's way; let's get back to the garden of Eden and live on top of the world! There is peace and everything we need and would need in the Kingdom of God.

Speak to be heard. Don't for a moment think your words and voice does not matter "It Does". Shout loud,be bold God created you for greatness! We are all unique and here to "showcase" our God given abilities... let's go create and bring out what's inside of you to give God the Glory!

Colossians 3:12-14 NKJV "Therefore, as the elect of God, holy and beloved, put on tender mercies, kindness, humility, meekness, longsuffering; bearing with one another, and forgiving one another, if anyone has a complaint against another; even as Christ forgave you, so you also must do. But above all these things put on love, which is the bond of perfection."

Colossians 4:3-4 NKJV "meanwhile praying also for us, that God would open to us a door for the word, to speak the mystery of Christ, for which I am also in chains, that I may make it manifest, as I ought to speak."

Colossians 3:17 NKJV "And whatever you do in word or deed, do all in the name of the Lord Jesus, giving thanks to God the Father through Him."

Feelings of Quitting

Have you ever had a feeling that you want to give up? How often have you had this feeling? What makes you feel like you want to give up? Do you want to give up on life? Do you want to give up on yourself? Do you want to give up on a relationship? Do you want to give up on a job? What is it that you want to give up? And what is it that you want to gain?

_____

_____

_____

Well I'm here to tell you that if you've ever wanted to give up on life you can give your life to Jesus right now. Let's ask God for salvation. Ask God for forgiveness of all the sins and let's repent.

Say these words out loud: "Lord, I come to you now just as I am, forgive me of all of my sins. Lord, I believe that Jesus died and rose again on the third day for my sins, come into my heart, live in me and through me from this day forward and I believe right now father God that I am your child, from this day forward I belong to you. Lord, direct me, guide me and I will never give up again in Jesus name Amen."

Romans 10:9-11 KJV "that if thou shalt confess with thy mouth the Lord Jesus, and shalt believe in thine heart that God hath raised him from the dead, thou shalt be saved. For with the heart man believeth unto righteousness; and with the mouth confession is made unto salvation. For the scripture saith, Whosoever believeth on him shall not be ashamed."

You have fallen out of agreement with giving up. You will no longer give up on anything. You will give it over to God and not give up. You totally give it over casting all my cares over to God. This means giving it all to God because God knows how to handle it. You must command the enemy to cease and desist from instigating the feeling of resignation or quitting in my life, in Jesus' name. Tell the enemy, your powers are broken now, in the name of Jesus.

Matthew 11:28-30 NKJV. "Come to Me, all you who labor and are heavy laden, and I will give you rest. Take My yoke upon you and learn from Me, for I am gentle and lowly in heart, and you will find rest for your souls. For My yoke is easy and My burden is light."

Matthew 11:28-30 AMP ""Come to Me, all who are weary and heavily burdened [by religious rituals that provide no peace], and I will give you rest [refreshing your souls with salvation]. Take My yoke upon you and learn from Me [following Me as My disciple], for I am gentle and humble in heart, and you will find rest (renewal, blessed quiet) for your souls. For My yoke is easy [to bear] and My burden is light.""

Solution:
God knows what it is; He knows where it came from. If it's a person God knows how to deal with that person. I pray you seek God. Seek the kingdom of God and his righteousness and all these things will be added onto you, no more giving up. Give it over to God once and for all, so be it unto you according to the word of God and your faith. God bless you.

Do you feel like you compare yourself to others?

Take a moment to describe your current situation, thoughts, feelings.

Write in the journal pages so you will be able to use this as reference in the future. This book is definitely interactive! I hope you will use this book as that tool with all of the strategies, principles and scriptures. Write down every time you're feeling the need to compare yourself to others (and why), then look at the word of God, gain hope again, so that we don't have to have these feelings wanting to compare yourself with man.

Ephesians 5:1-2 AMP "Therefore become imitators of God [copy Him and follow His example], as well-beloved children [imitate their father]; and walk continually in love [that is, value one another—practice empathy and compassion, unselfishly seeking the best for others], just as Christ also loved you and gave Himself up for us, an offering and sacrifice to God [slain for you, so that it became] a sweet fragrance."

3 John 1:11 AMP "Beloved, do not imitate what is evil, but [imitate] what is good. The one who practices good [exhibiting godly character, moral courage and personal integrity] is of God; the one who practices [or permits or tolerates] evil has not seen God [he has no personal experience with Him and does not know Him at all]."

Let's take the time and examine when we started to feel the need to compare yourself to others. Right now fall out of agreement with the feeling of comparison and all of those signs, symptoms and manifestations of comparison. Feelings of comparison are being destroyed and you are being delivered set free by the blood of Jesus Christ. I believe it for you right now, so be it unto you according to your faith. Lord we rejoice hallelujah that the feeling of comparison is removed, destroyed and thrown into the sea. You said whatsoever we bind on earth is bound in heaven. We bind comparison and lose the feelings of comfort, peace, feelings of being wanted and needed and the fact they are never alone again from this moment forward, my God send a blessing into their life.

Let them know you are with them. Lord we ask they imitate you not man.

Matthew 18:18-20 KJV "Verily I say unto you, Whatsoever ye shall bind on earth shall be bound in heaven: and whatsoever ye shall loose on earth shall be loosed in heaven. Again I say unto you, That if two of you shall agree on earth as touching anything that they shall ask, it shall be done for them of my Father which is in heaven. For where two or three are gathered together in my name, there am I in the midst of them."

Joshua 1:9 NKJV "Have I not commanded you? Be strong and of good courage; do not be afraid, nor be dismayed, for the LORD your God is with you wherever you go.""

What Has God been saying to you during this time of reading this book, day to day activities? I want you to be real transparent with yourself and know that there is help! God is here to help. Use the word of God (Bible) as your way to escape the negative feelings and watch God move on your behalf. God's word has power, God's word has life. God's word will deliver you out of each and every feeling of anxiety. God's word will bring you to where you need to be.

Solution:
Learn how to walk in faith with God. By walking in faith, remember faith comes by hearing, hearing by the word of God. Allow God to speak to you, (learn to hear God's voice, this is a process, keep that in mind).

Allow God to heal you from all brokenness, feelings of being battered, being misunderstood, anxiety, bad relationships, negativity, wickedness, generational curses, bad decisions, bad communication, bad character, lack of integrity, lack of self-control, self sabotage and fear.

Allow God to help with the emotional aspects of feeling tormented, hurt, abandonment, entrapment, the fear of no one cares, the fear of no one loves you and you are not being heard. Release the emotions, feelings and all aspects which go along with your deliverance in these areas. Do not do this alone, make sure you have an accountable person to help you with deliverance in these areas (someone trained).

In times of despair, the Word of God is an excellent source of hope and comfort. Scripture can give us a powerful reminder of God's love and our own potential for joy and greatness. Many people suffer from feelings of depression as life brings unwanted change and loss. Find encouragement and gratitude in these powerful Bible verses for depression. Scripture can be a powerful source of inspiration and healing, spiritually, mentally, and emotionally.

Do you care too much about what other people think?

Joshua 1:9 AMP "Have I not commanded you? Be strong and courageous! Do not be terrified or dismayed (intimidated), for the LORD your God is with you wherever you go.""

Job 11:18-19 AMP "Then you would trust [with confidence], because there is hope; You would look around you and rest securely. You would lie down with no one to frighten you, And many would entreat and seek your favor."

Proverbs 3:5-12 MSG "Trust GOD from the bottom of your heart; don't try to figure out everything on your own. Listen for GOD 's voice in everything you do, everywhere you go; he's the one who will keep you on track. Don't assume that you know it all. Run to GOD! Run from evil! Your body will glow with health, your very bones will vibrate with life! Honor GOD with everything you own; give him the first and the best. Your barns will burst, your wine vats will brim over. But don't, dear friend, resent GOD 's discipline; don't sulk under his loving correction. It's the child he loves that GOD corrects; a father's delight is behind all this."

1 Corinthians 5:9-13 GNT "In the letter that I wrote you I told you not to associate with immoral people. Now I did not mean pagans who are immoral or greedy or are thieves, or who worship idols. To avoid them you would have to get out of the world completely. What I meant was that you should not associate with a person who calls himself a believer but is immoral or greedy or worships idols or is a slanderer or a drunkard or a thief. Don't even sit down to eat with such a person. After all, it is none of my business to judge outsiders. God will judge them. But should you not judge the members of your own fellowship? As the scripture says, "Remove the evil person from your group.""

Do you dwell on things for no reason, constantly repeating scenarios over and over again in your mind?

Are you Worrying?

Do you want to be alone?

Do you rehearse what you are going to say to people?

Decrees

Decree: Proverbs 12:5 I decree that this day will be filled with strategic discernment and wise decisions

Decree: Isaiah 11:2 I decree this day I will be given access to supernatural might, strength, council, knowledge, and prophetic insight.

Decree: Psalms 2:8 NKJV "Ask of Me, and I will give You The nations for Your inheritance, And the ends of the earth for Your possession."

Decree: Luke 6:45 NKJV "A good man out of the good treasure of his heart brings forth good; and an evil man out of the evil treasure of his heart brings forth evil. For out of the abundance of the heart his mouth speaks."

Decree: I decree this is the last day you will have these feelings of doubt, discouragement, anger and loneliness.

Decree: I decree from this day forward you will handle all your life situations with positive words, thoughts and the word of God.

Decree: I decree you will live a life of peace.

Decree: I decree you are a overcomer and your faith is stronger than you can ever think or imagine.

Decree: I decree the favor of God is on your life and you will handle each challenge with God's power. You will speak to those situations and change them with your words.

Decree: I decree from this day forward you will not speak negativity and cause your circumstances to over take you ever again.

Decree: I decree you are blessed and your family is blessed. You are living a new lifestyle because of God.

Overcome Life Circumstances

Over the course of this book you read about several situations and solutions which are common to everyday life. This book was also interactive, you were able to write your feelings and take notes in the moment. The goal is to achieve and conquer one topic before going to the next (in the order you need most). Let's focus on getting help to cope, along with strategies and scriptures to live a better life.

If you can relate, just know you are about to change your trajectory on life. The goal was to provide solutions, from the Word of God, to help in several circumstances and situations we will go through in life. God will help you see things differently. Read with an open mind. Take notes, read and meditate on the scriptures. This will help conquer that situation that you are experiencing or know someone you can help from reading this book.

Once you read and meditate the scriptures in this book you will find peace, you will find healing, you will become stronger. You will find boldness, you will find faith over fear and you will find strength.

When you were weak you felt like giving up. You thought no matter what you said or did, your voice was not heard. Your voice is being heard. Keep speaking out. Stand up for what you believe in. Be bold. Realize there's no more torment, there's no more negativity. There is no more abandonment and you will no longer have to suffer or feel pain.

Romans 12:1-2 MSG "So here's what I want you to do, God helping you: Take your everyday, ordinary life—your sleeping, eating, going-to-work, and walking-around life—and place it before God as an offering. Embracing what God does for you is the best thing you can do for him. Don't become so well-adjusted to your culture that you fit into it without even thinking. Instead, fix your attention on God. You'll be changed from the inside out. Readily recognize what he wants from you, and quickly respond to it. Unlike the culture around you, always dragging you down to its level of immaturity, God brings the best out of you, develops well-formed maturity in you."

Proverbs 4:23-27 GNT "Be careful how you think; your life is shaped by your thoughts. Never say anything that isn't true. Have nothing to do with lies and misleading words. Look straight ahead with honest confidence; don't hang your head in shame. Plan carefully what you do, and whatever you do will turn out right. Avoid evil and walk straight ahead. Don't go one step off the right way."

Amos 9:13-15 MSG ""Yes indeed, it won't be long now." GOD 's Decree. "Things are going to happen so fast your head will swim, one thing fast on the heels of the other. You won't be able to keep up. Everything will be happening at once—and everywhere you look, blessings! Blessings like wine pouring off the mountains and hills. I'll make everything right again for my people Israel: "They'll rebuild their ruined cities. They'll plant vineyards and drink good wine. They'll work their gardens and eat fresh vegetables. And I'll plant them, plant them on their own land. They'll never again be uprooted from the land I've given them." GOD, your God, says so."

Jeremiah 33:2-3 MSG ""This is GOD's Message, the God who made earth, made it livable and lasting, known everywhere as GOD: 'Call to me and I will answer you. I'll tell you marvelous and wondrous things that you could never figure out on your own.'"

Matthew 28:18-20 GNT "Jesus drew near and said to them, "I have been given all authority in heaven and on earth. Go, then, to all peoples everywhere and make them my disciples: baptize them in the name of the Father, the Son, and the Holy Spirit, and teach them to obey everything I have commanded you. And I will be with you always, to the end of the age.""

James 5:13-16 GNT "Are any among you in trouble? They should pray. Are any among you happy? They should sing praises. Are any among you sick? They should send for the church elders, who will pray for them and rub olive oil on them in the name of the Lord. This prayer made in faith will heal the sick; the Lord will restore them to health, and the sins they have committed will be forgiven. So then, confess your sins to one another and pray for one another, so that you will be healed. The prayer of a good person has a powerful effect."

James 5:19-20 AMP "My brothers and sisters, if anyone among you strays from the truth and falls into error and [another] one turns him back [to God], let the [latter] one know that the one who has turned a sinner from the error of his way will save that one's soul from death and cover a multitude of sins [that is, obtain the pardon of the many sins committed by the one who has been restored]."

Proverbs 6:16-19 AMP "These six things the Lord hates; Indeed, seven are repulsive to Him: A proud look [the attitude that makes one overestimate oneself and discount others], a lying tongue, And hands that shed innocent blood, A heart that creates wicked plans, Feet that run swiftly to evil, A false witness who breathes out lies [even half-truths], And one who spreads discord (rumors) among brothers."

Scriptures To Meditate

Anger: Psalm 30:5

Fear: Psalm 23:4

Broken-hearted: Psalm 34:17-18

Hopeless: Isaiah 40:31, Isaiah 41:10

Anxiety: 1 Peter 5:7

Anxious: Philipians 4:6-7

Death: Romans, 6:23 Revelation 21:4

Hope and Deliverance: Philippians 4:13, John 10:10, Joshua 1:8-9, Proverbs 3:5-6 Matthew 6:33, Proverbs 3:5-6, Psalms 23:1, Philippians 4:19, Psalms 20:4, Amos 9:13-15 MSG, Proverbs 18:21, Romans 15:5, Philemon 1:7, Genesis 50:21, Deuteronomy 28, Genesis 1, 1 John 1

Affirmations

- ➔ I am the head not the tail
- ➔ I am victorious
- ➔ I am a game changer
- ➔ I am a Child of God
- ➔ I am walking by faith
- ➔ I am a overcomer
- ➔ I am love
- ➔ I am full of faith
- ➔ I am joy
- ➔ I am above only never beneath

Words of Encouragement to live successful

1. God must be first without question
2. God is your only source
3. God is ready to help you in every area of my life if you allow God to be God
4. Pray daily (especially to start your day)
5. Praise God Always
6. Faith in God and know without faith it is impossible to please God
7. Have a firm foundation and relationship with God (intimacy)
8. Doing things God's way is the only way
9. Bible is here to find solutions to everyday situations
10. Remember you matter to God
11. God loves you

Conclusion

Trust in the word of God. If you are saying I don't know God yet, you will know God and have a better relationship after studying and reading this devotional. Your mindset will be changed and you will learn to trust again. You will learn to love yourself and no longer have self-doubt! You will no longer feel worthless, you will no longer feel lost. You will no longer feel like you have to struggle. You will no longer feel bound. All shackles will be removed, you will see single eyed! You will look straight ahead. You will no longer look backwards, you will start leaving all the past behind.

God has a purpose and plan for everyone's life. God has not forgotten you. God is love. God is here. Use faith over fear! Have an intimate relationship with God and tell God how we are feeling. One hundred percent open, let's be honest, let's be real, let's be very transparent, with yourself, let's be honest, let's open up and allow God to heal all of your brokenness.

I encourage you, whatever you're going through, there is nothing too hard for God.

Whatever you are about to face, God already knows, tell God. God will give you the answers, you need to be still, in a peaceful quiet place to hear his voice.

Author Sharron Downs

Sharron Downs - Consultant, Life Coach, Mentor, Motivational Speaker and Influencer. Servitude is my passion. I have a passion to help those with depression, loneliness, low self esteem, trauma, difficult feelings and other mental Instability.

I have a BS in Psychology, Leadership and Life Coach Certificates. I've discovered how important speaking positive words are in every area of my life. My podcast "Sharron Daily Inspirations" on platforms where you listen to podcasts. I have a passion to encourage, motivate and inspire others. I'm a leader and influencer. I have something great to share with others, my voice.

Books written and published by Sharron Downs

"Change Your World With Words -Add Value To Every Area Of Your Life" ISBN-13 979-8725146905 ASIN B08ZD6TK8T

"21 Strategies To Overcome Mental Instability: With The Words You Speak" ISBN-13 979-8728031918 ASIN B08ZW3186N

"Beauty For Ashes Book 1 (3 Book Series) - 21 Day Devotional" ISBN-13 979-8731480451 ASIN B091GN7271

"Beauty For Ashes Devotional: Discover Your Value" (Beauty for Ashes Devotional: 7 Day Devotional) ISBN-13 979-8732724219 ASIN B091J98QV8

"Joy and Gladness" (Beauty For Ashes Devotional: 7 Day Devotional) ISBN-13 979-8732804287 ASIN B091NPVTD8

"Renew Restore Refresh: 27 Day Devotional" ISBN-13 979-8733179094 ASIN B0924CY24W

"Decree A Thing: Speak And Command" Change ISBN-13 979-8509544644 ASIN B095GP9HNP

"Dominate Emotional Instabilities: Break Free- Gain Control of your mind" ISBN-13 979-8516343889 ASIN B096LPS1Q5

"Beauty For Ashes: 30 Day Journal" ISBN-13 979-8512556382 ASIN B096LYJWR6

"Change Your World With Your Words second Edition" ISBN-13 979-8510183726 ASIN B095MKPHFF

"Words Carry Power: Speak Words of Faith" ISBN-13 979-8524636355 ASIN B097C2VM8S

"Overcome Life Circumstances: With The Word of God" (currently being published)

Notes:

Write down your thoughts, feelings and put a date next to it so when you are delivered from it you will know how long it was since you confessed the cycle has now been broken. Remember this is a process. This book is an interactive tool to help with life's circumstances. The objective is to recognize you have a need and be ready for change, God's way.

_____

_____

_____

_____

www.ingramcontent.com/pod-product-compliance
Lightning Source LLC
Chambersburg PA
CBHW070645220526
45466CB00001B/307